SELF-CARE FOR THE DEMENTIA CAREGIVER

A SURVIVAL GUIDE WITH ESSENTIAL TIPS TO AVOID CAREGIVER BURNOUT

RENEE PHILLIPPI

As I wrote Dementia for Caregivers, I realized many books like it focus on caring for the *patient*. That's when I decided to create this comprehensive guide for _you_, the caregiver, to help you navigate your caregiving journey and cope with the challenges you'll face. This guide will give you the tools to take the best care of yourself.

If you've found this book helpful, please leave a review on Amazon so that others may find it, too.

CONTENTS

"Caregiving is not for the weak; it requires strength, resilience, and a boundless heart."

— DONNA CARDILLO

INTRODUCTION

Caregiving is a truly noble and selfless endeavor, and I want to commend you for embarking on this journey to care for someone with dementia. Your presence and dedication will undoubtedly make a significant difference in their life. However, we must acknowledge that the road ahead may present significant challenges. It's crucial to approach this task with a gentle and comforting mindset, both for the person you will be caring for and for yourself.

Dementia is a complex condition that affects not only memory but also cognition and behavior. It can be disorienting, frustrating, and emotionally taxing for the individual and their caregiver. There may be times when communication becomes problematic when the person you care for may not recognize you or may exhibit unpredictable behavior. These moments can be heart-wrenching, but please remember that they do not reflect your worth or your capabilities as a caregiver.

Being patient with yourself and the person you're caring for is essential. Celebrate the small victories and cherish the moments of clarity. Educate yourself about dementia and seek support from professionals and support groups. They can provide guidance, resources, and a safe space to express your feelings and concerns.

This journey will require physical, emotional, and mental strength. Practice self-care, engage in activities that bring you joy, and reach out for help when needed. It's not selfish to take care of yourself—*it's necessary to maintain your well-being.*

Lastly, know that you are not alone. There's a vast community of caregivers who understand and share your experiences. They can provide practical advice, encouragement, and overall emotional support. By connecting with others, you can find solace and learn valuable strategies for navigating the challenges that lie ahead.

Remember, these recommendations are general guidelines. You should consult a registered dietitian or healthcare professional who can provide personalized advice based on your specific health conditions, medications, and goals.

In addition to proper nutrition, there are other factors to consider for maintaining your well-being as a caregiver. The following chapters will give you specific ways to overcome the challenges of being a caregiver and suggest ways to care for yourself.

Taking care of your well-being is crucial to ensure you have the physical and mental capacity to provide the best care for your loved one with dementia. Following these guidelines and prioritizing self-care can support your health and well-being throughout your caregiving journey.

Self-Care: Prioritize self-care activities that help you relax and rejuvenate. Engage in hobbies you enjoy, practice mindfulness or meditation, take breaks when needed, and get sufficient sleep.

Stress Management: Find healthy ways to manage stress. This can include deep breathing exercises, practicing mindfulness, engaging in relaxation techniques, or seeking support from a therapist or counselor.

Social Support: Stay connected with friends, family, and support groups. Surrounding yourself with a support network can provide emotional support, understanding, and an opportunity to share experiences and advice.

Time Management: Establish a routine and prioritize tasks. Create a schedule that allows time for you to take breaks and for self-care activities. Delegate responsibilities to others when possible and avoid overextending yourself.

Seek Help: Remember that it is not a sign of weakness to ask for help. Reach out to family, friends, or professional caregivers to provide assistance and respite care when needed.

> "You gain strength, courage, and confidence by every experience in which you really stop to look fear in the face. You must do the thing which you think you cannot do."
>
> — ELEANOR ROOSEVELT

First, before we review your plan for caring for yourself, we'll discuss a few things you should consider and have in place as you start this journey.

PRE-PLANNING

Developing a comprehensive care plan is crucial when caring for someone with dementia. It helps ensure that their needs are met and provides structure and guidance for the caregiver and the person with dementia. The following are essential steps to consider as you start this journey.

Assess the person's needs: Start by assessing the specific needs of the person with dementia. Consider their physical, cognitive, emotional, and social requirements. Consider their strengths, limitations, and personal preferences. This assessment will form the foundation of the care plan.

Involve healthcare professionals: Consult with healthcare professionals, such as doctors, geriatric specialists, or dementia care specialists. They can provide valuable insights, guidance, and medical advice. They'll help you understand the progression of dementia, anticipate future challenges, and suggest appropriate interventions.

Establish a routine: Create a consistent daily routine that provides structure and familiarity. People with dementia often find comfort in routine. Determine regular times for meals, activities, and personal care. Consistency helps reduce confusion and agitation and makes it easier to manage their needs.

Ensure safety and adapt to the environment: Identify potential hazards and make necessary modifications to create a safe environment. Install handrails, remove clutter, use locks or alarms on doors and windows, and secure dangerous items. Consider adaptations like grab bars, nonslip mats, or specialized equipment to support their mobility and daily activities.

Address medical and medication management: Ensure that the person you're caring for receives appropriate medical care. Schedule regular check-ups and screenings. Organize their medication regimen using pill organizers or digital reminders. Communicate with healthcare professionals about any changes in their condition and report any concerns promptly.

Develop communication strategies: As dementia progresses, communication becomes more challenging. Develop effective communication strategies that accommodate their changing abilities. Use clear, simple language, speak calmly and slowly, and allow time for processing. Look for non-verbal cues like facial expressions and gestures.

Encourage social engagement and meaningful activities: Socialization and engagement will enhance their quality of life. Plan activities that align with their interests and abilities. These may include puzzles, music therapy, arts and crafts, or reminiscing. Maintain connections with family, friends, and support groups to prevent social isolation. Keep in touch with friends and family members.

Emotional and self-care support: Provide emotional support not only to the person with dementia but also to yourself as the caregiver. Seek respite care when needed to prevent burnout. Engage in self-care activities, connect with support networks, and consider joining caregiver support groups to share experiences and gain insights from others in similar situations.

Regular evaluation and adjustment: Regularly evaluate the effectiveness of the care plan and make necessary adjustments. Dementia is a progressive condition, and care needs will change over time. Stay flexible and adapt the plan to accommodate new challenges, evolving abilities, and emerging needs.

THE 7 STAGES OF DEMENTIA

Here are the 7 stages of dementia and what to expect as your patient/loved one progresses through the disease.

Stage 1 - No Impairment

The absence of any visible symptoms characterizes the initial stage of dementia, but the disease has already begun to affect the brain. Amyloid PET scans can help diagnose dementia, revealing signs of amyloid clumps up to two decades before symptoms occur (Bhandari, 2021).

Stage 2 - Slight Cognitive Decline

The second stage, "Slight Cognitive Decline," is characterized by the onset of memory or cognitive confusion, which may go unnoticed. While the patient's social and organizational skills remain intact, symptoms such as misplacing keys, forgetting familiar names, or the location of frequently used objects may occur. These are innocent memory lapses that can happen to anyone.

Stage 3 - Mild Cognitive Decline

In stage three of dementia, mild cognitive decline becomes more noticeable, drawing the attention of those around the patient. Memory lapses now pertain to recent events or newly learned information. Individuals may also struggle with word retrieval or misuse of words, which can be a new experience for them. Working memory is one of the first abilities to decline, leading to difficulties forming and retaining new short-term memories. The inability to concentrate and pay attention can also impact work performance.

Even routine tasks such as taking medication or attending appointments may become more challenging due to impaired planning and organizational skills. However, because symptoms can persist for several years before progressing to the next stage, dementia is not typically diagnosed yet.

Stage 4 - Moderate Cognitive Decline

Stage four is typically when a diagnosis of dementia is made as cognitive impairments become more apparent. Symptoms in earlier stages become more severe, while new ones may also arise. For instance, long-term memory loss may become more frequent, and the patient may struggle to remember events from their past. Social and behavioral skills also decline, leading to withdrawal, apathy, and irritability. Patients may deny or refuse to acknowledge their condition. Due to the worsening of cognitive and behavioral skills, the individual may require part-time care and support from their family.

Stage 5 - Moderately Severe Cognitive Decline

Stage five is characterized by a severe cognitive decline that requires a full-time caregiver to assist with daily activities. Patients may experience more frequent episodes of confusion, feeling lost, and forgetting the names of relatives. Although long-term memory

remains intact, critical aspects of daily life may be impaired, such as preparing meals or getting dressed, necessitating special assistance. However, basic needs like toilet use may still be carried out independently.

Stage 6 - Severe Cognitive Decline

Stage six is commonly known as "middle dementia." The patient experiences severe cognitive decline and worsening physical difficulties at this stage. They require complete assistance from a caregiver, even for basic tasks like toileting and showering. Although they might still remember episodes from their past life, it is a highly debilitating phase where they come to terms with their condition and acknowledge the amount of care they need. The patient experiences mood changes due to irregular sleep patterns, including agitation, anger, and depression.

Stage 7 -Very Severe Cognitive Decline

In the seventh and final stage of dementia, patients experience the most severe physiological limitations, making it the most challenging stage for caregivers to manage. The patient's ability to control bowel movements and perform basic tasks, such as swallowing and speaking, is significantly compromised. Speaking ability is almost entirely lost, and the patient might only be able to say a few disconnected words. Physical movements become slower due to the dopamine deficiencies experienced at this stage. Swallowing difficulties can lead to recurring pneumonia caused by aspiration, posing a severe risk to the patient's life, given their compromised immune system.

ANGER, GRIEF, GUILT AND LOSS

Caring for a person with dementia can evoke many complex emotions for caregivers, including anger, guilt, grief, and loss. Understanding and effectively dealing with these emotions is essential for maintaining your emotional well-being while providing care. Here's a guide to help you navigate and cope with these challenging emotions:

Anger:

Anger is a common emotion experienced by caregivers due to the frustrations and challenges of caring for a loved one with dementia. It's essential to acknowledge and manage anger constructively.

Recognize triggers: Identify situations, behaviors, or circumstances that trigger your anger. Awareness can help you anticipate and prepare for these triggers.

Take a break: When anger arises, step away from the situation temporarily. Take deep breaths, go for a walk, or engage in a calming activity to regain composure.

Express your frustration: Share your feelings with a trusted friend, support group, or therapist. They can provide empathy, understanding, and guidance on healthy ways to cope with anger. Journaling is an excellent way to express your thoughts if you're uncomfortable sharing them.

Practice self-care: Participate in activities that help you relax and release tension, such as exercise, meditation, or hobbies. Prioritizing self-care will reduce stress and anger.

Guilt:

Guilt is a common emotion experienced by caregivers, stemming from a sense of not doing enough or feeling responsible for the challenges faced by their loved ones. Here are some ways to cope with guilt.

Seek support: If you have feelings of guilt, share these with a support group or counselor who can provide reassurance, guidance, and a fresh perspective.

Accept limitations: Recognize that it is impossible to control or fix every aspect of the dementia journey. Understand that you are doing your best within the given circumstances.

Celebrate small victories: Acknowledge and appreciate the positive moments and efforts you make in caregiving. Focus on the difference you are making, no matter how small.

Practice self-compassion: Treat yourself with understanding and kindness. Remind yourself that caregiving is challenging, and sometimes it is okay to feel overwhelmed. Take breaks and prioritize self-care without guilt.

Grief and Loss:

Caring for a loved one with dementia often involves witnessing the gradual loss of their cognitive and functional abilities. Here are some ways to cope with grief and loss.

Acknowledge your feelings: Allow yourself to experience and express your emotions related to the losses associated with dementia. Permit yourself to grieve.

Seek emotional support: Connect with others who have experienced similar losses, such as support groups or online communities. Talking to people who understand can provide comfort and validation.

Educate yourself about dementia: Understanding the progression of the disease can help you navigate the stages of grief more effectively.

Being informed about the disease can also help you adjust expectations and find ways to provide appropriate care.

Celebrate moments of connection: Focus on finding joy in the present moment. Cherish the times when your loved one shows glimpses of recognition or when you share meaningful interactions.

Seek professional help: Remember, it's normal to experience anger, guilt, grief, and loss as a caregiver, and you may experience all these emotions many times throughout the stages. However, if these emotions become overwhelming or interfere with your daily life, seeking professional help is advisable. A therapist or counselor can provide tailored guidance and support for your specific situation.

Self-care is not a luxury but a necessity. By taking care of yourself physically and emotionally, you're building resilience that will enable you to navigate the caregiving journey with greater strength and endurance, ultimately benefiting you and the person you are caring for. You've seen this several times already, and it is repeated many more times in this book: ***Self-care must be one of your priorities***. Let's get to it, shall we?

YOUR PLAN FOR SELF CARE

1

DIET, NUTRITION AND EXERCISE

P roper nutrition is essential for caregivers caring for someone with dementia. Maintaining a balanced diet to support your physical and mental well-being is vitally important. The following recommendations will help guide you toward making healthy food choices:

Tips for a Balanced and Nutrient-Rich Diet

Include a variety of fruits and vegetables: These are rich in vitamins, minerals, antioxidants, and fiber. Aim to fill half your plate with colorful fruits and vegetables at each meal. Choose whole grains options like whole wheat bread, brown rice, and whole grain cereals. They provide more fiber and nutrients compared to refined grains. Include lean proteins such as fish, chicken, turkey, legumes, tofu, and low-fat dairy products. Protein is vital for muscle maintenance and repair.

Incorporate healthy fats like avocados, nuts, seeds, and olive oil. These fats support brain health and provide sustained energy.

Effects of Caffeine

Moderate your caffeine intake. Caffeine can temporarily boost energy, but too much can lead to jitters, anxiety, disrupted sleep patterns, and increased heart rate.

Consider timing – Avoid consuming caffeinated beverages close to bedtime, as it may interfere with sleep quality. Opt for decaffeinated options later in the day.

Effects of Sugar

Limit added sugars. Too much intake of added sugars can lead to energy crashes, weight gain, and an increased risk of chronic diseases. Read food labels to find hidden sources of added sugars in processed foods and beverages.

Choose natural sources of sweetness: Instead of relying on refined sugars, satisfy your sweet tooth with naturally sweet foods like fruits. Fruits provide essential vitamins, minerals, and fiber along with sweetness.

Effects of Dehydration

Stay hydrated. Dehydration can lead to fatigue, cognitive decline, decreased focus, and other health issues. Drink water regularly throughout the day and increase your intake during warmer weather or when physically active.

Monitor fluid intake: Keep track of your fluid intake and aim to drink at least 8 cups (64 ounces) of water daily. If you struggle with drinking plain water, try adding fruits or herbs for added flavor.

Exercise:

Prioritize physical activity. Engaging in regular exercise is crucial for maintaining your physical and mental well-being. Physical activity helps reduce stress, improves mood, boosts energy levels, and enhances cognitive function. Choose activities you enjoy: Find activities that you genuinely enjoy, whether it's walking, swimming, dancing, gardening, or yoga. This will increase adherence and make exercise more enjoyable.

Aim for at least 2 hours per week. Strive for at least 2 hours of moderate-intensity exercise, such as brisk walking, spread throughout the week. Add strength training exercises to maintain muscle mass and bone health if possible.

Break it into smaller sessions – If finding a continuous block of time for exercise is challenging, break it down into shorter sessions. For example, three 10-minute walks can still provide benefits.

Consult a healthcare professional if you have any underlying health conditions or concerns, consult with a healthcare professional before starting a new exercise program.

Caregiving is exhausting. Even when you take care of yourself, exercise, and cut out harmful things in your diet, there will be days when you are not hungry or just too tired to cook. For that reason, I've listed 20 days of healthy, quick, and easy recipes for breakfast, lunch, dinner, desserts, and snacks.

2

RECIPES

Breakfast

1. **Greek Yogurt Parfait**: Add berries, a handful of nuts, and a drizzle of honey to Greek yogurt. Top with chia seeds.
2. **Veggie Scrambled Eggs**: Scramble 2 eggs with diced bell peppers, onions, spinach, and a sprinkle of low-fat cheese.
3. **Oatmeal with Fruits**: Cook oats in almond milk, top with sliced fruits like bananas, berries, and a sprinkle of cinnamon.
4. **Avocado Toast**: Top a slice of whole wheat bread with mashed avocado. Sprinkle with chia seeds.
5. **Protein Smoothie**: Blend spinach, banana, blueberries, Greek yogurt, and a scoop of protein powder with some ice.
6. **Whole Grain Cereal with Almond Milk**: Choose a high-fiber, low-sugar cereal. Top with some berries or a banana.
7. **Quinoa Porridge**: Cook quinoa in almond milk. Sweeten with mashed banana and top with berries.
8. **Peanut Butter Banana Toast**: Spread natural peanut butter on whole wheat bread top with sliced banana.
9. **Fruit & Nut Yogurt**: Mix Greek yogurt with your choice of fruit and a small handful of nuts.

10. **Spinach & Tomato Frittata**: Beat eggs, add sautéed spinach and tomatoes to a pan, and cook until set.
11. **Chia Seed Pudding**: Mix chia seeds with almond milk a drizzle of honey, and let it sit overnight. Top with fresh fruits in the morning.
12. **Veggie Omelette**: Mix eggs with chopped bell peppers, tomatoes, onions, and spinach. Cook on a pan.
13. **Almond Butter Smoothie**: Blend banana, almond butter, almond milk, and a handful of spinach.
14. **Blueberry Quinoa**: Cook in almond milk, top with blueberries, a drizzle of honey, and a sprinkle of cinnamon.
15. **Whole Grain Pancakes**: Use whole grain flour to make pancakes, top with fresh fruits and a drizzle of honey.
16. **Protein-Packed Oatmeal**: Cook oats with milk, stir in protein powder, and top with nuts and berries.
17. **Breakfast Burrito**: Fill a tortilla with black beans, scrambled eggs, salsa, and avocado.
18. **Mango Smoothie Bowl**: Blend frozen mango with Greek yogurt. Top with granola and fresh berries.
19. **Baked Avocado Egg**: Bake an egg in a halved avocado. Sprinkle with salt and pepper.
20. **Overnight Oats with Fruits**: Mix oats, milk, chia seeds and refrigerate overnight. Top with fresh fruits in the morning.

Lunch

1. **Chicken and Avocado Salad**: Mix grilled chicken, sliced avocado, mixed greens, cherry tomatoes, and cucumber. Dress with olive oil and lemon juice.
2. **Turkey Wrap**: Whole wheat tortilla, lean turkey, lettuce, tomato, and avocado. Roll and cut into portions.
3. **Baked Salmon with Quinoa and Broccoli**: Bake salmon and broccoli in olive oil, salt, and pepper. Serve with cooked quinoa.
4. **Lentil Soup**: Sauté onion, carrots, celery, garlic in olive oil, add lentils and vegetable broth, simmer.

5. **Quinoa Salad**: Mix cooked quinoa, mixed greens, cherry tomatoes, cucumber, and feta cheese. Dress with lemon juice and olive oil.
6. **Tofu Stir Fry**: Stir-fry tofu with colorful veggies. Add soy sauce, garlic, and ginger.
7. **Vegetarian Tacos**: Fill whole grain tortillas with black beans, salsa, lettuce, tomatoes, and avocado.
8. **Greek Salad**: Mix tomatoes, cucumbers, feta, olives, and red onion. Dress with olive oil and lemon juice.
9. **Avocado Egg Salad**: Mix boiled eggs with avocado instead of mayo. Serve on whole grain bread or lettuce.
10. **Chickpea Salad**: Mix chickpeas, cucumber, tomatoes, onions, and feta. Dress with olive oil and lemon juice.
11. **Tuna Salad Wrap**: Mix tuna with chopped celery, onion, and Greek yogurt. Fill a whole-grain tortilla.
12. **Egg Salad Sandwich**: Mix boiled eggs with Greek yogurt, mustard, salt, and pepper. Serve on whole-grain bread.
13. **Quinoa Stuffed Peppers**: Stuff bell peppers with cooked quinoa, black beans, corn, tomatoes, and bake.
14. **Vegetable Sushi Rolls**: Roll sushi with avocado, cucumber, carrots, and brown rice.
15. **Chicken Caesar Salad**: Mix grilled chicken, lettuce, whole grain croutons, sprinkle with low-fat Caesar dressing.
16. **Broccoli Soup**: Blend cooked broccoli, onions, garlic, a dash of cream or milk, and add vegetable broth—season with salt and pepper.
17. **Tofu & Veggie Kebabs**: Skewer tofu, bell peppers, zucchini, cherry tomatoes. Grill.
18. **Whole Grain Pizza with Veggies**: Top a whole grain pizza base with tomato sauce, low-fat cheese, and lots of veggies. Bake.
19. **Fish Tacos**: Fill whole grain tortillas with grilled fish, cabbage slaw, and avocado.
20. **Spinach and Strawberry Salad**: Mix fresh spinach, strawberries, and almonds. Dress with balsamic vinaigrette.

Dinner

1. **Chicken Stir Fry**: Stir-fried chicken with colorful veggies. Add soy sauce, garlic, and ginger.
2. **Whole Wheat Pasta with Spinach and Cherry Tomatoes**: Cook pasta, sauté spinach and tomatoes in garlic and olive oil. Combine.
3. **Turkey Chili**: Cook lean ground turkey; add beans, tomatoes, peppers, onion, and chili powder. Simmer.
4. **Baked Cod with Roasted Veggies**: Bake cod with lemon and herbs. Serve with roasted colorful veggies.
5. **Vegetable Curry**: Sauté onions, garlic, ginger, curry powder, colorful veggies and coconut milk. Simmer.
6. **Grilled Chicken with Sweet Potato and Asparagus**: Grill chicken, roast sweet potato, and asparagus in olive oil.
7. **Stuffed Bell Peppers**: Stuff bell peppers with tomatoes, rice, and cooked lean ground beef or turkey. Bake.
8. **Shrimp and Broccoli Stir Fry**: Stir-fry shrimp and broccoli in garlic and ginger. Add soy sauce.
9. **Bean and Vegetable Tacos**: Fill whole grain tortillas with refried beans, colorful veggies, and salsa.
10. **Chicken Salad Sandwich**: Mix boiled eggs with Greek yogurt, mustard, salt, and pepper. Add canned or steamed chicken. Serve on whole-grain bread.
11. **Chicken Caesar Salad**: Mix grilled chicken, lettuce, whole grain croutons, sprinkle with low-fat Caesar dressing.
12. **Broccoli Soup**: Blend cooked broccoli, onions, and garlic with vegetable broth season with salt and pepper.
13. **Tofu & Veggie Kebabs**: Skewer tofu, bell peppers, zucchini, cherry tomatoes. Grill.
14. **Whole Grain Pizza with Veggies**: Top a whole grain pizza base with tomato sauce, low-fat cheese, and lots of veggies. Bake.
15. **Fish Tacos**: Fill whole grain tortillas with grilled fish, cabbage slaw, and avocado.
16. **Spinach and Strawberry Salad: Mix fresh spinach, strawberries, and** almonds. Dress with balsamic vinaigrette.

17. **Pesto and Tomato Panini:** Spread a tablespoon of pesto on a slice of bread. Add tomato slices and mozzarella cheese. Top with another slice of bread and heat in a panini press or good in a pan until the bread is toasted or the cheese is melted.
18. **Caprese Avocado Salad:** Chop 2 avocados and 2 tomatoes. Add pieces of mozzarella cheese and basil leaves. Drizzle with a balsamic glaze and season with salt and pepper.
19. **BLT Salad Wraps:** Chop bacon and tomatoes and mix with mayonnaise. Spoon into a romaine lettuce leaf and close with a toothpick if necessary.
20. **Avocado Toast with Egg:** Top a piece of toast with a ripe, mashed avocado, and top with an egg—season with salt and pepper.

Snacks

1. **Celery with Peanut Butter and Raisins**: Spread celery sticks with peanut butter and top with raisins.
2. **Greek Yogurt with Berries and Honey**: Mix Greek yogurt with berries and drizzle with honey.
3. **Hummus and Veggie Sticks**: Serve colorful veggie sticks with hummus.
4. **Apple Slices with Almond Butter**: Spread almond butter on apple slices.
5. **Cherry Tomatoes with Mozzarella**: Skewer cherry tomatoes and mozzarella balls. Drizzle with olive oil and balsamic vinegar.
6. **Baked Kale Chips**: Tear kale into pieces bake with olive oil, and a pinch of salt until crisp.
7. **Cucumber Sandwiches**: Use cucumber slices instead of bread; fill with turkey and low-fat cheese.
8. **Mixed Nuts**: A handful of unsalted mixed nuts.
9. **Fruit Salad**: Mix your choice of fruits and squeeze a little lime juice on top.
10. **Roasted Chickpeas**: Roast chickpeas with olive oil, salt, and your choice of spices until crispy.

11. **Avocado Salsa**: Mix diced avocado, tomato, onion, cilantro, and lime juice. Serve with whole-grain tortilla chips.
12. **Hard-Boiled Eggs**: Boil eggs and sprinkle with a pinch of salt.
13. **Almond Butter & Banana Toast**: Spread almond butter on whole-grain toast and top with sliced banana.
14. **Greek Yogurt with Honey and Nuts**: Mix Greek yogurt with a small handful of nuts and drizzle with honey.
15. **Cherry Tomatoes Stuffed with Tuna**: Hollow out cherry tomatoes, fill with tuna mixed with Greek yogurt.
16. **Veggie Chips**: Thinly slice carrots, beets, sweet potatoes, bake until crisp.
17. **Homemade Trail Mix**: Mix nuts, seeds, dried fruits, and dark chocolate chips.
18. **Fresh Fruit**: Simply enjoy a piece of fresh fruit for a nutritious snack.
19. **Cottage Cheese with Berries**: Mix cottage cheese with a handful of berries.
20. **Edamame**: Steam edamame sprinkle with a pinch of salt.

Desserts

1. **Dark Chocolate Covered Strawberries**: Melt dark chocolate, dip strawberries, and let cool.
2. **Fruit Salad with Honey and Lime**: Mix your choice of fruits, drizzle with honey, and squeeze a little lime juice.
3. **Baked Apple with Cinnamon**: Bake an apple, drizzle with honey, and sprinkle with cinnamon.
4. **Banana Ice Cream**: Blend frozen banana slices until creamy; add a little vanilla extract.
5. **Fruit Kebabs**: Skewer chunks of your favorite fruits.
6. **Yogurt and Berry Popsicles**: Blend Greek yogurt and berries and freeze in popsicle molds.
7. **Dark Chocolate and Almond Clusters**: Melt dark chocolate, stir in almonds, drop spoonfuls onto wax paper, let cool.
8. **Chia Seed Pudding**: Stir almond milk and a little honey, then add chia seeds. Let sit in the fridge to thicken.

9. **Greek Yogurt with Mixed Berries and Dark Chocolate Chips**: Mix Greek yogurt with berries and a small handful of dark chocolate chips.
10. **Baked Pear with Honey and Walnuts**: Bake a pear, drizzle with honey, and top with walnuts.
11. **Fruit Salad with Mint**: Mix your fruit top with chopped mint.
12. **Greek Yogurt with Cinnamon and Apples**: Mix Greek yogurt with diced apples and sprinkle with cinnamon.
13. **Banana & Berry Sorbet**: Blend frozen bananas and berries until creamy.
14. **Oatmeal Cookies**: Make cookies with oats, bananas, and dark chocolate chips. Bake.
15. **Peach & Raspberry Crisp**: Top peaches and raspberries with oats, almonds, and honey. Bake.
16. **Apple & Almond Butter Sandwiches**: Slice apple into rounds and spread with almond butter.
17. **Frozen Greek Yogurt Bark**: Spread Greek yogurt on a baking sheet and top with berries and nuts. Freeze.
18. **Roasted Cinnamon Plums**: Halve plums, sprinkle with cinnamon, and roast until soft.
19. **Frozen Grapes**: Freeze grapes for a refreshing dessert.
20. **Dark Chocolate Dipped Orange Slices**: Melt dark chocolate, dip orange slices, and let cool.

INFUSED WATER RECIPES

You, too, should make sure you stay hydrated. Try these recipes to increase water intake.

1. **Cucumber and Mint**: Slice cucumber and a few mint leaves. Add to water and let infuse.

2. **Strawberry and Basil**: Slice strawberries and a few basil leaves. Add to water and let infuse.

3. **Lemon and Ginger**: Slice lemon and ginger. Add to water and let infuse.

4. **Pineapple and Mint**: Dice pineapple and add some mint leaves. Add to water and let infuse.

5. **Orange and Blueberry**: Slice oranges and add some blueberries. Add to water and let infuse.

6. **Apple Cinnamon**: Slice apples and add a few cinnamon sticks. Add to water and let infuse.

7. **Blueberry Lime**: Add some blueberries and sliced lime. Add to water and let infuse.

8. **Blackberry Mint**: Add some blackberries and mint leaves. Add to water and let infuse.

9. **Lemon Raspberry**: Add sliced lemon and raspberries. Add to water and let infuse.

10. **Pomegranate Lime**: Add pomegranate seeds and sliced lime. Add to water and let infuse.

---

50 SELF-CARE IDEAS FOR CAREGIVERS

Here are some activities for self-care.

1. Take a warm bath with soothing bath salts or oils.
2. Engage in regular exercise, such as yoga, walking, or swimming.
3. Practice meditation or deep breathing exercises.
4. Set aside time for reading a book or listening to an audiobook.
5. Learn a new hobby or skill that you find enjoyable.
6. Schedule regular outings or activities with friends.
7. Take short breaks throughout the day to relax and recharge.
8. Keep a gratitude journal and write down things you are thankful for.
9. Get a massage or practice self-massage techniques.
10. Attend a support group for caregivers to connect with others who understand your experiences.
11. Practice mindfulness by focusing on the present moment and letting go of worries about the past or future.
12. Engage in creative activities such as painting, drawing, or playing a musical instrument.
13. Watch your favorite movie or TV show that brings you joy.

14. Spend time in nature, whether it's going for a walk in the park or sitting in a garden.
15. Listen to uplifting or calming music that helps you relax.
16. Treat yourself to a spa day or a professional beauty treatment.
17. Cook or bake a favorite recipe as a form of creative expression and enjoyment.
18. Take a day trip to a place you find peaceful or inspiring.
19. Engage in volunteer work or community service that aligns with your interests and values.
20. Practice gentle stretching or yoga poses to release tension and promote flexibility.
21. Enjoy a cup of herbal tea or a soothing beverage of your choice.
22. Practice self-compassion and offer yourself kindness and understanding during challenging times.
23. Set boundaries and say no when needed to protect your own time and energy.
24. Spend quality time with a pet, whether it's playing, petting, or cuddling with them.
25. Go for a scenic drive or take a walk in a new neighborhood.
26. Engage in aromatherapy using essential oils that promote relaxation, such as lavender or chamomile.
27. Engage in a digital detox and limit screen time for a specific period each day.
28. Plan a weekend getaway or a short vacation to rejuvenate and recharge.
29. Practice progressive muscle relaxation to release tension in your body.
30. Engage in a hobby that allows you to be creative, such as knitting, gardening, or woodworking.
31. Treat yourself to a favorite dessert or indulge in a special treat.
32. Practice self-reflection and journal about your own personal growth and journey as a caregiver.
33. Practice forgiveness towards yourself and others to let go of resentment and find peace.
34. Watch or listen to comedy shows or podcasts to laugh and uplift your mood.

35. Engage in a digital hobby or learn something new online, such as photography or playing a musical instrument.
36. Visit a museum or art gallery to appreciate and immerse yourself in art and culture.
37. Engage in progressive relaxation exercises to relax your body and mind.
38. Spend time with loved ones who provide support and positive energy.
39. Engage in deep cleaning or organizing activities to create a sense of order and clarity.
40. Practice visualization techniques to imagine peaceful and positive scenarios.
41. Attend a yoga or meditation class to deepen your practice and connect with a supportive community.
42. Take a leisurely walk in nature and connect with the healing power of the outdoors.
43. Attend a spiritual or religious gathering that aligns with your beliefs and provides a sense of community.
44. Enjoy a picnic in a beautiful outdoor setting.
45. Engage in a hobby such as playing a musical instrument, painting, dancing, or anything that brings you joy.
46. Practice self-care rituals, such as taking time for skincare, grooming, or pampering yourself.
47. Engage in expressive writing, such as journaling or writing poetry.
48. Set aside time for quiet reflection and introspection.
49. Seek professional counseling or therapy to prioritize your mental and emotional well-being.
50. Keep a journal to express your thoughts, emotions, and experiences.

5

STRESS MANAGEMENT

Laughter is a powerful tool that can positively impact the brain and help caregivers relax while caring for someone with dementia. It has been shown to have numerous benefits, both physical and psychological. Understanding how it affects the brain can provide valuable insights into its potential to alleviate stress, improve mood, and enhance overall well-being. Here's an explanation of the effects of laughter and how it can help caregivers relax:

It stimulates the release of endorphins. Endorphins are natural chemicals in the brain that promote feelings of pleasure and reduce pain. These act as natural mood elevators, helping to counteract stress and create a sense of well-being. As a result, laughter can help reduce stress, tension, and anxiety, allowing caregivers to relax and unwind.

Engaging in laughter limits the release of cortisol, a stress hormone. It also increases the production of dopamine and serotonin, neurotransmitters associated with positive emotions. The release of these "feel-good" chemicals can help reduce stress and anxiety, promoting a sense of calm and relaxation in caregivers.

Furthermore, it has been found to enhance the functioning of the immune system. It boosts the production of antibodies and activates immune cells, increasing their effectiveness in combating illnesses and infections. A robust immune system is vital for caregivers, as it helps protect against common ailments and ensures their overall well-being.

Laughter also promotes social connection and strengthens relationships. When caregivers share moments of laughter with their loved ones with dementia, it can create a sense of connection and improve the quality of their interactions. This can bridge communication gaps and engage with the person emotionally, fostering a deeper sense of understanding and empathy.

In addition to its social benefits, it profoundly impacts mood regulation. It can lift spirits, foster a positive outlook, and counteract feelings of sadness, frustration, or helplessness. Caregivers often face emotionally challenging situations, and laughter can serve as a coping mechanism, allowing them to experience moments of joy and light amidst the difficulties they encounter.

When we laugh, we engage in deep breathing, which increases oxygen intake and improves blood flow. This oxygenation positively impacts brain function, promoting mental clarity and alertness. By increasing oxygen levels, laughter supports overall brain health and cognitive functioning.

Beyond its physical and psychological effects, laughter can serve as a temporary diversion from the challenges and difficulties of caregiving. It offers a break from the stressors, providing a light-hearted and enjoyable experience. By redirecting focus and shifting perspective, laughter can help caregivers momentarily escape the pressures of their responsibilities and find moments of respite.

Engaging in laughter regularly can also improve resilience in the face of adversity. It helps caregivers maintain a positive mindset, adapt to challenging situations, and find moments of joy and humor even in difficult circumstances. Cultivating resilience is crucial for caregivers as it allows them to bounce back from setbacks and maintain their well-being.

Incorporating laughter into your caregiving routine can be achieved through various means. Share humorous stories, memories, or anecdotes with your loved one with dementia. Watch comedy movies, TV shows, or stand-up performances together. Engage in playful activities or games that elicit laughter. Spend time with friends, family, or support groups who bring positivity and humor into your life.

By embracing laughter as a relaxation tool, caregivers can experience the benefits of reduced stress, improved mood, enhanced social connection, and overall well-being. Laughter is a natural and accessible resource that caregivers can utilize to care for themselves while providing compassionate care to their loved ones with dementia.

6

RELAXATION TECHNIQUES

As a caregiver of someone with dementia, it's important to prioritize your well-being and find ways to relax and reduce stress. Caring for a loved one with dementia can be emotionally and physically demanding, and taking time for yourself is essential to maintain your health. Incorporating relaxation techniques into your daily routine can help you manage stress, improve your overall well-being, and provide a sense of calm amidst the challenges you may face. Here are several relaxation techniques that you can consider:

Breathing Exercises for Stressful Moments:

During moments of high stress or when you feel overwhelmed, take a few deep breaths to help calm your nervous system. Inhale deeply through your nose while counting to four, hold the breath for a moment, and then exhale slowly through your mouth. Repeat this process several times, focusing on the breath and allowing yourself to regain composure and a sense of calm.

Progressive Muscle Relaxation:

Start by tensing and then releasing each muscle group in your body, one at a time. Begin with your toes, curling them tightly, then release the tension, allowing them to relax completely. Move gradually through your body, tensing and relaxing your legs, abdomen, arms, shoulders, and facial muscles. Focus on the sensations of tension leaving your body and enjoy the feeling of relaxation as each muscle group releases.

Guided Imagery:

Close your eyes and imagine yourself in a peaceful, serene environment, such as a tranquil beach or calming forest.

Engage your senses by visualizing the details of the scene, including the sights, sounds, smells, and textures. Take time to immerse yourself in the imagery, allowing it to transport you to a place of relaxation and tranquility. Guided imagery can be enhanced using pre-recorded audio guides or apps that provide calming visualizations and soothing music.

Mindfulness Meditation:

Find a quiet space where you can sit comfortably and without distractions. Focus your attention on your breath, the sensations in your body, or a chosen object of focus. If your mind wanders, gently redirect your attention back to your chosen focal point without judgment. Practice mindfulness for a few minutes daily, gradually increasing the duration.

Yoga and Stretching:

Engage in gentle yoga poses or stretching exercises to promote relaxation and release tension in your body. Start with simple stretches,

such as reaching for the sky, touching your toes, or gentle twists.

Consider following a yoga video or attending a local class specifically designed for relaxation and stress reduction. Focus on the breath and the sensations in your body as you move through each pose, allowing your mind to calm.

Music Therapy:

Listen to calming and soothing music that helps you relax and unwind.

Choose instrumental or classical pieces with slow rhythms and melodic tunes. Create a playlist of your favorite calming songs or explore pre-made relaxation playlists on streaming platforms. Take a few moments to close your eyes, focus on the music, and let it wash away stress and tension.

Engaging in Hobbies or Creative Activities:

Participate in activities that bring you joy and help you unwind, such as painting, gardening, knitting, or playing a musical instrument.

Engaging in hobbies allows you to focus on something enjoyable and provides a sense of accomplishment and relaxation.

Make time for activities that bring you happiness and allow you to recharge.

Journaling:

Write your thoughts, feelings, and experiences in a journal or diary. Journaling can help you process emotions, gain perspective, and release stress. Set aside a few minutes daily to reflect and write freely, without judgment or concern for grammar or style.

You can also use journaling to express gratitude, jotting down what you are thankful for each day. Check the table of contents to find guided journaling pages in this book.

The 4-7-8 Breathing Technique to Help Fall Asleep

Dr. Andrew Weil developed this technique. Sit or lie down. Exhale through your mouth, then inhale through your nose as you count to four silently. Hold that breath for seven seconds, then exhale through your mouth with force. Start out with only 4 breaths in the beginning. Increase to 8 breaths as you practice this technique over a few days or week.

Positive Affirmations

Introduce or reinforce a more positive mindset by reciting positive affirmations. Check the table of contents to find 31 affirmations in this book to repeat.

Taking Time for Yourself:

Carve out dedicated time for self-care and relaxation regularly.

Whether taking a bath, reading a book, going for a walk, or just enjoying a cup of tea, prioritize activities that rejuvenate and recharge you.

Remember, each person is unique, and different relaxation techniques may resonate differently with individuals. Explore these techniques and find what works best for you. Incorporating relaxation practices into your routine will benefit your well-being and enhance your ability to provide care and support to your loved one with dementia.

7

TEN WAYS TO PREVENT CAREGIVER BURNOUT

Caregiver burnout is a genuine concern when caring for a person with dementia. Still, there are strategies you can implement to lessen its effects and prioritize your well-being. Here are ten ways to accomplish this:

1. Stay Organized: Get into a daily routine or use tools like calendars and reminder apps to manage your caregiving responsibilities. Being organized can reduce feelings of chaos.
2. Ask for and accept help: Don't hesitate to ask for and accept help from others—delegate tasks like running errands or meal preparation to lighten your workload. Remember, you don't have to do it all alone.
3. Prioritize self-care: Make time for activities that recharge and rejuvenate you. Engage in hobbies, exercise regularly, practice mindfulness or meditation, and get enough sleep. Taking care of yourself is essential for your well-being.
4. Set realistic expectations: Be realistic about what you can accomplish in a day. Understand that there will be limitations and challenges. Celebrate small victories and be gentle with yourself when things don't go as planned.

5. Establish boundaries: Learn to set boundaries and say "no" when necessary. It's essential to recognize your limits and not overextend yourself. Protect your physical and emotional energy by prioritizing your needs.

6. Practice stress management techniques: Incorporate stress management techniques into your daily routine. Deep breathing exercises, yoga, or calming music can help you relax and manage stress.

7. Take breaks and respite: Arrange regular breaks and respite care to give yourself time to recharge. Taking breaks is essential to prevent burnout, whether it's a short walk, a few hours off, or a weekend getaway.

8. Educate yourself: Learn more about dementia to understand the challenges and develop effective caregiving strategies. Knowledge empowers you to make informed decisions and provide better care.

9. Stay connected: Maintain social connections outside of caregiving. Make time for friends, hobbies, and activities that bring you joy. Talk to friends and invite them over when you can't leave your loved one. Staying connected with others will help prevent feelings of isolation and provide a support network.

10. Seek professional help: If you are consistently overwhelmed or experiencing signs of depression or anxiety, consider seeking professional help. A therapist or counselor can provide valuable guidance and support.

Remember, taking care of yourself is not selfish—it is essential for providing quality care to your loved one. By implementing these strategies and seeking support, you can lessen the effects on caregiver burnout and maintain your well-being throughout your caregiving journey.

However, it's important to recognize that caregiver burnout is a serious issue, and these suggestions may need to be revised for everyone. If you find yourself in a situation where you are struggling significantly or feeling overwhelmed, it's crucial to reach out for professional help and support.

TIME MANAGEMENT

Establishing a routine and effectively prioritizing tasks is crucial for caregivers caring for someone with dementia. It helps create structure, maintain consistency, and ensure that both the caregiver and the person with dementia have their needs met. Here's a comprehensive guide on establishing a routine, creating a schedule that allows for breaks and self-care activities, and delegating responsibilities when possible.

Understand the Needs and Preferences:

Observe the person with dementia to identify their patterns, preferences, and times of day when they are most alert or agitated.

Consider their routines, hobbies, and interests, and try to incorporate those into your schedule.

Create a Daily Plan:

Start by outlining the essential activities, such as meals, medication management, personal care, and appointments. Allocate specific time slots for each activity, considering the person's energy levels and attention span. Incorporate engaging and enjoyable activities, such as outings, hobbies, puzzles, or listening to music, to promote social interaction and mental stimulation.

Prioritize Tasks:

Identify the most critical tasks and prioritize them based on urgency and importance.

Break down larger tasks into smaller, manageable steps to make them more achievable.

Consider the individual's preferences and prioritize activities that bring them comfort, joy, and a sense of normalcy.

Allocate Time for Breaks and Self-Care:

Schedule regular breaks for yourself throughout the day to rest and recharge. Use this time to engage in activities promoting relaxation and self-care, such as reading, walking, or practicing mindfulness.

Be realistic about the time you need for breaks and ensure they are built into the schedule.

Delegate Responsibilities:

Identify tasks that can be delegated to others, such as family members, friends, or hired caregivers. Delegate responsibilities that do not require your direct involvement, such as housekeeping, grocery shopping, or transportation.

Communicate your needs to your support network and ask for help when necessary. Don't hesitate to reach out for assistance and accept help when offered.

Seek Respite Care:

Consider utilizing respite care services, which provide temporary relief for caregivers. This can be through professional caregivers who come to the home or through respite care facilities.

Respite care allows you to take a break from caregiving responsibilities, ensuring you have time to rest, rejuvenate, and attend to your needs.

Flexibility and Adaptability:

Understand that flexibility is vital when caring for someone with dementia. Be prepared for routine changes and be adaptable to their needs and preferences as they fluctuate.

Modify the schedule as necessary based on the person's condition, mood, or energy levels. Stay attuned to their cues and adjust the plan accordingly.

Communication and Collaboration:

Communicate the daily routine to the person with dementia using simple language. Use visual aids, such as a schedule or calendar, to help them understand and anticipate activities.

Involve the person with dementia in decision-making to the extent they are capable. Offer choices whenever possible to maintain a sense of autonomy and control.

Utilize Technology and Tools:

Explore technological aids, such as reminder apps, alarms, or electronic calendars, to help manage appointments, medication schedules, and daily routines. Use adaptive devices or tools that simplify tasks and promote independence for the person with dementia, reducing the burden on the caregiver. Don't underestimate the value of joining Facebook groups for dementia caregivers.

Regular Evaluation and Adjustments:

Regularly assess the effectiveness of the routine and schedule. Note any challenges or areas that require improvement. Be open to making adjustments and refinements based on the evolving needs of the person with dementia and your well-being. Remember, establishing a routine and prioritizing tasks is a dynamic process. It may take time to find a schedule that works best for both the person with dementia and the caregiver. Be patient, flexible, and compassionate with yourself and the person you're caring for. Prioritizing breaks and self-care activities is essential to prevent burnout and ensure you can provide the best care possible.

9

TEN SIGNS THAT INDICATE YOU MAY NEED ASSISTANCE

Remember, recognizing the signs of caregiver burnout and asking for help is not a sign of weakness; it is a testament to your commitment to providing the best care for your loved one. Taking care of your well-being ensures that you can continue to be an effective and compassionate caregiver.

1. Exhaustion and fatigue: Feeling constantly physically and emotionally drained despite adequate rest.
2. Overwhelming stress: Feeling overwhelmed and unable to cope with the demands of caregiving.
3. Neglected personal well-being: Neglecting your own physical and mental health, skipping meals, or not finding time for self-care activities.
4. Social isolation: Withdrawing from social activities and relationships due to caregiving responsibilities.
5. Lack of time for other responsibilities: Struggling to meet personal and household obligations or maintain a job.
6. Difficulty managing behavior changes: Feeling challenged in managing your loved one's behavioral symptoms associated with dementia, such as agitation or aggression.

7. Frequent accidents or safety concerns: Noticing an increase in accidents or safety risks for you and the person with dementia.
8. Declining physical health: Experiencing a decline in physical health due to the strain of caregiving.
9. Emotional distress: Feeling constant sadness, anxiety, anger, or resentment related to your caregiving role.
10. Lack of respite: Finding it difficult to take breaks or find time for yourself, leading to continuous caregiving without relief.

If you notice these signs, seeking help and support is essential. Don't hesitate to contact healthcare professionals, support groups, or family and friends. Consider respite care options to give yourself a break and recharge. Utilize community resources or hire a professional caregiver to assist you.

10

GUIDED JOURNALING PAGES

As you navigate the challenges ahead, exploring journaling as a means of self-reflection and self-care may be beneficial. These pages serve as a safe space to express and document your emotions, allowing you to observe your personal growth and the positive impact of implementing self-care practices.

Use the following pages with prompts to begin journaling.

Today's Moments:

_____

_____

A time today when I felt proud:

_____

_____

Something my loved one enjoyed today:

_____

_____

A challenging moment and how I addressed it:

_____

_____

_____

How did I feel today as a caregiver?

_____

_____

_____

One self-care activity I did for myself today:

_____

_____

_____

Tomorrow's Goals:

_____

_____

Today's Moments:

_____

_____

A time today when I felt proud:

_____

_____

Something my loved one enjoyed today:

_____

_____

A challenging moment and how I addressed it:

_____

_____

_____

How did I feel today as a caregiver?

_____

_____

_____

One self-care activity I did for myself today:

_____

_____

_____

Tomorrow's Goals:

_____

_____

Today's Moments:

_____

_____

A time today when I felt proud:

_____

_____

Something my loved one enjoyed today:

_____

_____

A challenging moment and how I addressed it:

_____

_____

_____

How did I feel today as a caregiver?

_____

_____

_____

One self-care activity I did for myself today:

_____

_____

_____

Tomorrow's Goals:

_____

_____

Today's Moments:

_____

_____

A time today when I felt proud:

_____

_____

Something my loved one enjoyed today:

_____

_____

A challenging moment and how I addressed it:

_____

_____

_____

How did I feel today as a caregiver?

_____

_____

_____

One self-care activity I did for myself today:

_____

_____

_____

Tomorrow's Goals:

_____

_____

Today's Moments:

_____

_____

A time today when I felt proud:

_____

_____

Something my loved one enjoyed today:

_____

_____

A challenging moment and how I addressed it:

_____

_____

_____

How did I feel today as a caregiver?

_____

_____

_____

One self-care activity I did for myself today:

_____

_____

_____

Tomorrow's Goals:

_____

_____

Today's Moments:

_____

_____

A time today when I felt proud:

_____

_____

Something my loved one enjoyed today:

_____

_____

A challenging moment and how I addressed it:

_____

_____

_____

How did I feel today as a caregiver?

_____

_____

_____

One self-care activity I did for myself today:

_____

_____

_____

Tomorrow's Goals:

_____

_____

Today's Moments:

_____

_____

A time today when I felt proud:

_____

_____

Something my loved one enjoyed today:

_____

_____

A challenging moment and how I addressed it:

_____

_____

_____

How did I feel today as a caregiver?

_____

_____

_____

One self-care activity I did for myself today:

_____

_____

_____

Tomorrow's Goals:

_____

_____

Today's Moments:

_____

_____

A time today when I felt proud:

_____

_____

Something my loved one enjoyed today:

_____

_____

A challenging moment and how I addressed it:

_____

_____

_____

How did I feel today as a caregiver?

_____

_____

_____

One self-care activity I did for myself today:

_____

_____

_____

Tomorrow's Goals:

_____

_____

Today's Moments:

_____

_____

A time today when I felt proud:

_____

_____

Something my loved one enjoyed today:

_____

_____

A challenging moment and how I addressed it:

_____

_____

_____

How did I feel today as a caregiver?

_____

_____

_____

One self-care activity I did for myself today:

_____

_____

_____

Tomorrow's Goals:

_____

_____

Today's Moments:

_____

_____

A time today when I felt proud:

_____

_____

Something my loved one enjoyed today:

_____

_____

A challenging moment and how I addressed it:

_____

_____

_____

How did I feel today as a caregiver?

_____

_____

_____

One self-care activity I did for myself today:

_____

_____

_____

Tomorrow's Goals:

_____

_____

Today's Moments:

_____

_____

A time today when I felt proud:

_____

_____

Something my loved one enjoyed today:

_____

_____

A challenging moment and how I addressed it:

_____

_____

How did I feel today as a caregiver?

_____

_____

_____

One self-care activity I did for myself today:

_____

_____

Tomorrow's Goals:

_____

_____

Today's Moments:

_____

_____

A time today when I felt proud:

_____

_____

Something my loved one enjoyed today:

_____

_____

A challenging moment and how I addressed it:

_____

_____

_____

How did I feel today as a caregiver?

_____

_____

_____

One self-care activity I did for myself today:

_____

_____

_____

Tomorrow's Goals:

_____

_____

Today's Moments:

_____

_____

A time today when I felt proud:

_____

_____

Something my loved one enjoyed today:

_____

_____

A challenging moment and how I addressed it:

_____

_____

_____

How did I feel today as a caregiver?

_____

_____

_____

One self-care activity I did for myself today:

_____

_____

_____

Tomorrow's Goals:

_____

_____

Today's Moments:

_____

_____

A time today when I felt proud:

_____

_____

Something my loved one enjoyed today:

_____

_____

A challenging moment and how I addressed it:

_____

_____

_____

How did I feel today as a caregiver?

_____

_____

_____

One self-care activity I did for myself today:

_____

_____

_____

Tomorrow's Goals:

_____

_____

11

POSITIVE AFFIRMATIONS FOR CAREGIVERS

A ffirmations are positive, empowering statements that you repeat. Instead of letting doubts or negative self-talk dominate your thoughts, affirmations remind you of your strength, purpose, and capacity for love and patience. By repeating these affirmations, you'll overcome negative thoughts and dispel self-doubt. This can help reduce stress and help affirm your value and worth.

Try repeating some or all of the following affirmations every morning or whenever you're experiencing negative thoughts.

1. I make a difference in their life.
2. I bring comfort, even if it is not apparent.
3. I am strong and capable.
4. I can do this!
5. Today, I will cherish the moments of clarity.
6. I am not alone in this journey.
7. The essence of my loved one is still here, even if it's hidden.
8. I am the definition of love and understanding.
9. Today, I will forgive myself for my imperfections.
10. My presence is reassurance.
11. We will always be connected by the heart.

12. Today, I will focus on love and empathy.
13. I will make beautiful memories, even during the challenges.
14. I will be patient today, even when it feels challenging.
15. I know I'm doing the best I can in this moment.
16. My love is stronger than any memory that is lost.
17. I am a harbor of safety in a sea of the unknown.
18. My love and care is shown by my compassion.
19. I can see the soul within, beyond the disease.
20. I learn and grow stronger in my role every day.
21. Every challenge is a testament to my dedication.
22. Today's challenges will be tomorrow's memories of strength.
23. I make a difference, one day at a time.
24. Today, I choose to see the light in every part of darkness.
25. I will connect with gentle words and kind gestures.
26. Today, I will sow seeds of comfort and security.
27. I will embrace the beauty in unexpected moments today.
28. In every challenge, I will find the lesson of grace.
29. Today, I choose kindness, patience, and understanding.
30. I am resilient.
31. The love I give will return to me in countless ways.

12

BLANK JOURNALING PAGES

YOUR PLAN FOR SELF CARE

YOUR PLAN FOR SELF CARE

_____

_____

_____

_____

_____

_____

_____

_____

_____

_____

_____

_____

_____

_____

_____

_____

_____

_____

_____

_____

_____

_____

YOUR PLAN FOR SELF CARE

_____

_____

_____

_____

_____

_____

_____

_____

_____

_____

_____

_____

_____

_____

_____

_____

_____

_____

_____

_____

_____

_____

CONCLUSION

W ith the information and insights provided, you're now equipped with the necessary tools and understanding to prioritize your own well-being while embarking on this journey alongside your loved one with dementia.

Remember, your dedication as a caregiver is admirable, but it's equally important to extend that same level of care and compassion to yourself. By nurturing your needs and well-being, you can ensure you can provide the best care possible for your loved one.

Embrace this opportunity to embark on a journey of self-discovery, self-care, and personal growth. You are not alone, and a community of support is available to you every step of the way. Trust in your abilities, be kind to yourself, and remember that even small acts of self-care can make a significant difference in your overall well-being.

"The heart of a caregiver is a unique blend of tenderness, compassion, resilience, and strength."

— ANONYMOUS

RESOURCES

Centers for Disease Control and Prevention https://www.cdc.gov/aging/aginginfo/alzheimers.htm

Dementia Society of America https://www.cdc.gov/aging/aginginfo/alzheimers.htm

Lewy Body Dementia Association https://www.lbda.org/

Support for Vets with Dementia https://www.va.gov/GERIATRICS/pages/Alzheimers_and_Dementia_Care.asp

National Aphasia Association https://www.aphasia.org/aphasia-resources/dementia/

Center Watch - Clinical Trials https://www.centerwatch.com/directories/1068-useful-resources/listing/2641-dementia-society-of-America

Parkinson and Movement Disorder Alliance https://www.pmdalliance.org/
Michael J Fox Foundation for Parkinson's Research https://www.michaeljfox.org/

Parkinson's Foundation https://www.parkinson.org/

International Parkinson and Movement Disorder Society https://www.movementdisorders.org/MDS/Resources/Patient- Education.htm

Memory Cafe Directory https://www.memorycafedirectory.com/ Dementia Friendly America https://www.dfamerica.org/

Centers for Medicare and Medicaid Services https://www.cms.gov/

Compare Nursing Home and Health Providers https://www.medicare.gov/care-compare/

Alzheimer's Association https://www.alz.org/

Other books by this author:

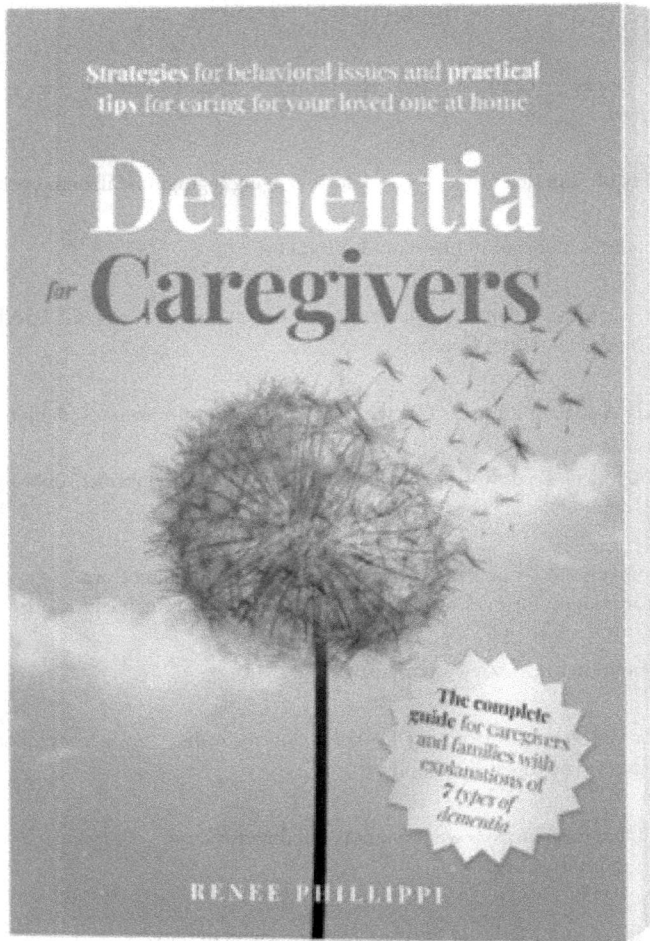

Strategies for behavioral issues and practical tips for caring for your loved one at home

Dementia
for Caregivers

The complete guide for caregivers and families with explanations of 7 types of dementia

RENEE PHILLIPPI

www.ingramcontent.com/pod-product-compliance
Lightning Source LLC
Chambersburg PA
CBHW060517280326
41933CB00014B/2996